MW01069855

1

Essential Oil for Beginners

The Ultimate Essential Oils Guide for

Beginners

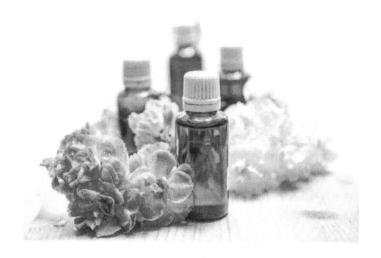

Essential Oil for Beginners

The Ultimate Essential Oils Guide for Beginners

Includes History, Benefits, Household Uses, Safety Tips, Essential Oils for Headaches, Sleep, Anxiety, and Other Ailments

Olivia Banks

Copyright © 2018 by Olivia Banks

All rights reserved. No part of this publication may be
reproduced, distributed, or transmitted in any form or by
any means, including photocopying, recording, or other
electronic or mechanical methods, without the prior
written permission of the publisher, except in the case of
brief quotations embodied in critical reviews and certain
other non-commercial uses permitted by copyright law.

CAC Publishing

Olivia Banks

ISBN: 978-1-948489-12-6

Contents

Introduction

Plant based oils and aromas have been used since time immemorial by thousands of communities and cultures across the world. They were even considered valuable products which could be used to: purchase luxurious items, pay dowry, settle disputes and offered as a gift to the gods; rivaling the likes of gold and silver. They have stood the test of time. The process of extracting oils from plants is something that has transformed and today it is much more efficient and cost effective. There is not much of a difference in terms of how various essential oils were being used in the past versus how they are being used today. The only change we've seen is that more uses have been developed for these oils.

The world of essential oils is so vast that more and more oils continue to be discovered as their usage expands. Often times it can be quite overwhelming as a beginner looking to get into this industry. *"The Ultimate Guide to Essential Oils"* aims to provide you with all the necessary information about essential oils in a detailed and easy to understand fashion. This book will help you identify the basic and most popular oils and their uses while gradually introducing you to more composite oils. You will learn how to create custom blends that work for you as well as the best ways to introduce their wonderful effects to your body. I hope that you will have fun and enjoy reading this book!

Chapter 1: History and Evolution

What are Essential Oils?

Essential oils are natural aromatic compounds found in the seeds, bark, stems, roots, flowers and other parts of plants gathered from around the world. While it is true they can be very fragrant, essential oils are extremely therapeutic. These natural oils are usually distilled from plants and are used most commonly for aroma therapy

Generally, these oils can be used in three different ways. The first one is known as **diffusion**. It involves the spreading of a type of oil into the air using a special device called a diffuser. Diffusers might be electrical devices you plug in or a sort of cup that holds essential oils and is then heated by a candle to diffuse the smell throughout the air.

One of the other ways to use an essential oil is the **topical** application meaning you are applying an essential oil right to your skin. However, some oils shouldn't be applied directly to your skin at all; while some should be diluted with other oils like coconut oil before it even touches your skin.

The other method is referred to as **ingestion**. Some people ingest essential oils whether taking a straight drop in their mouth or in a glass of water or even in their cooking. Extreme caution should be taken when ingesting essential oils as some can be very toxic. You should research and / or consult your doctor before ingesting any essential oil.

Essential oils are considered a dietary aide and provide vitality and well-being. They contain multifaceted naturally occurring compounds which makes them unique. These unique molecules allow essential oils to work with all the cells and tissues in the body.

It has been estimated that essential oils can be as much as 70 times more effective than dried herbs. As a matter of fact, one drop of peppermint is as potent as 28 cups or more of peppermint tea. Essential oils are immediately reactive in the body because their chemical structures are already in their most usable form.

Not all essential oils are alike. To be safe and effective, they must be pure and free from any alterations that would reduce their therapeutic benefit and their life sustaining properties.

In order to be most effective and beneficial, essential oils must be sourced in their native and often indigenous habitat.

Brief History and Timeline

Throughout history, people have used many forms of plant medicine; especially essential oils. Many believe that the Egyptians were the first to discover the benefits and therapeutic effects of these oils. As a matter of fact, essential oils were considered to be very valuable. Grave robbers often left the gold and jewels in the tombs and took only the oil. Over time, other cultures used essential oils for a variety of therapeutic treatments.

Many cultures around the world have used essential oils or aromatic oils as they were once called. While it may be quite difficult to pin point exactly when the use of essential oils began spreading, research into ancient civilization and societies have been able to give us a picture of just how popular these oils were in the past. Now, let us briefly examine some evidence of early use of essential oils.

France

So far, the earliest evidence of use of essential oils by human beings was found in a place called Lascaux in the Dordogne region of France. This region is covered by an extensive network of complex caves. Inside some of these caves are cave paintings that suggest the use of herb oils and medicinal plants in everyday life of the residents of that area. Carbon dating estimates the cave paintings to be at least 20,000 years old; meaning they were carved as far back as 18,000 B.C.E.

Egypt

Evidence along with recorded history of early Egyptians regarding use of essential oils is much more concrete. As far back as 5,000 B.C.E, Egyptians used aromatic oils and ointments for various purposes. As a matter of fact, at the time, they had made a name for themselves as experts in cosmetology and ointments; with their star herbal concoction called "Kyphi". It was used as medicine, incense and perfume and was made from a mixture of 16 ingredients.

The average citizen of Egypt used perfumed oils, resins, balsams, aromatic vinegars, spices and scented barks in their daily lives. Oils were extracted from plants to make pastes, powders, ointments, medicinal cakes as well as pills. Also used extensively during this period were: ashes and smoke from garlic, aniseed, grapes, watermelon and onion. However, it is worth noting that the use of aromatic oils was a privilege that was only reserved for priests; particularly at the height of the Egyptian Empire. It was viewed as a divine product that could only be handled by representatives of the gods.

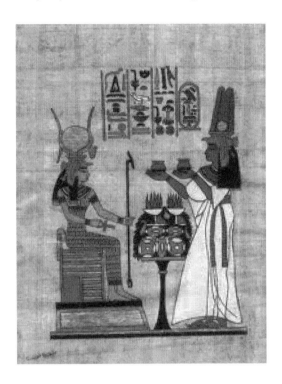

To get a clearer picture, each deity had their own specific fragrance while the pharaohs also had their own special oils for various uses such as meditation and war. For purposes of preserving dead bodies, usually pharaohs and other high ranking royal family members, the early Egyptians used aromatic gums derived from cedar and myrrh. Evidence of their use has been traced to mummies found in recent times.

However, Egypt didn't always manufacture all the oils they used; they imported some – particularly cedar and cypress oils.

China

Use of essential oils in China was first recorded between the years 2697 B.C.E and 2597 B.C.E. Perhaps the most important piece of evidence with regards to this subject is the well documented journal called *"The Yellow Emperor's Book of Internal Medicine"* written during the reign of Emperor Huang Ti. Regarded as the oldest surviving medical book in China, it contains information on more than 300 herbs and their medicinal applications. To date, classic practitioners of eastern medicine still use it for research information.

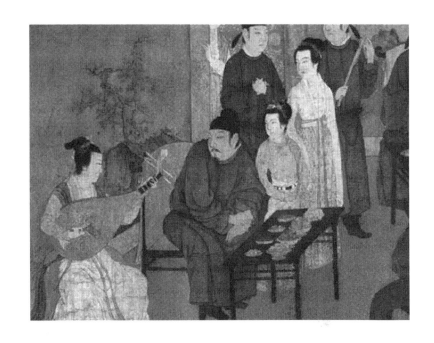

India

A 3,000-year old branch of traditional Indian medicine known as *"Ayur Veda"* is very popular for its extensive use of essential oils. With an archive of more than 700 substances such as: myrrh, cinnamon, ginger and sandalwood in Vedic medicinal literature, traditional Indian medicine is regarded as one of the most comprehensive forms of traditional and alternative medicine.

Ayur Veda has been tried and tested thanks to its success in helping contain the spread of the Bubonic Plague by replacing some antibiotics that weren't working.

The use of aromatic oils was not just limited to medicinal purposes. Spiritual and philosophical outlook was also a major sphere of life for ancient Indians and these oils played a key role here as well.

Greece

Ancient Greek medicine (400 B.C.E to 500 B.C.E) contains a blend of ancient Egyptian medicine practices and the traditional Indian Ayur Veda, both of which are founded on essential oils. In ancient Greece, Hippocrates was commonly known as the *"Father of Medicine"*. He once said, *"I believe that a daily aromatic bath followed by a scented massage will promote good health"*. Under his advisement, soldiers often carried into battles ointments of myrrh to fight off infections. His literature contains documented effects of more than 300 plants such as marjoram, cumin, thyme and saffron.

Hippocrates was drawn to Ayurvedic medicine after Greek soldiers encountered it during their journeys with Alexander the Great and found it to be harmonious with Greek medicine. One of his many noble accomplishments was when he saved Athens from a deadly plague by fumigating the city with aromatics. To understand just how much of an influence and impact Hippocrates' work has had, all doctors today are required to take what is known as the *'Hippocratic Oath'*.

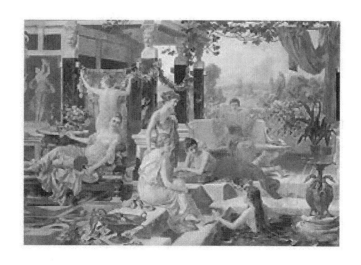

Europe

Use of essential oils for medicinal and spiritual purposes by the 14th Century was quite extensive across Europe. For instance, the knights during the crusades passed on knowledge of herbal medicine they had picked up from their travels in the Middle East. Also recorded in history books is how burning frankincense and pine in the streets during the Bubonic Plague helped contain the outbreak. More recently, in 1928, a French chemist called René-Maurice Gattefossé published the book "Aromatherapie" which describes in detail various essential oils and their healing capabilities.

Modern trends toward a more holistic approach to self-care and growing scientific validation of alternative health practices are driving a rediscovery of the profound health benefits of essential oils.

Evolution

The most well-known and recorded method of ancient extraction of essential oils is perhaps the method coined by ancient Egyptians. Now, since the process of using steam for distillation to extract essences was not invented back then, they had to use other techniques. One such method is called Enfleurage. It involves saturation of layers of fat with perfume by steeping flowers in the fat and replacing them when their perfume was spent. The flower petals are placed on a layer of glass that is spread with a layer of fat. What happens is that the volatile oil in the petals diffuses into the fat which is then collected and then oil is extracted from it using alcohol. This method is not used today because it is very expensive and time consuming. However, it worked for the ancient Egyptians and other ancient communities as well.

Today, the most commonly used methods for extraction of essential oils are:

- Steam distillation method
- Solvent extraction method

- Carbon dioxide extraction method
- Maceration process

Religious References of Essential Oils

There is a lot of reference to essential oils made in The Bible – both the Old and New Testament. Specifically mentioned are: myrrh, myrtle, frankincense, fir, spikenard, cinnamon and cedar wood. A well-known reference is one made regarding the birth of the child Christ during which he received gifts in the form of frankincense, myrrh and gold. Another reference of essential oils is made when Moses received the formula for holy anointing oil which included: olive oil, clove, cinnamon and myrrh.

The Holy Quran also makes reference to certain plants and plant extractions which were to be used as directed by Prophet Muhammad for medicinal purposes. They include: Onions (Basal), Hina (Henna), Grapes (Inab), Camphor (Kafoor), Date palm (Khajoor), Sweet Basil (Rehan), Figs (An-jeer) and many more.

Spiritual use of aromatic oils was not just limited to Christians and Muslims. As mentioned in the previous section, they were also used by ancient Egyptians, Jews, Indians as well as traditional African societies for spiritual purposes.

The World of Aromatherapy: Brief Introduction and Facts

Aromatherapy is the use of plant materials and plant oils to positively affect mood, psychological and / or physical well-being. In simple terms it comes down to: you smell nice things and it makes you feel good.

Aromatherapy has been around for thousands of years and basically involves your smell sense and different natural substances as a beneficial aid to your health and mental faculties.

So how is aromatherapy performed? Well, this is how:

✓ Directly inhaling essential oils through the nostrils from the bottle or off a cloth

✓ By diffusing one or a combination of essential oils into the surrounding air

✓ By rubbing the oils directly onto your skin

✓ By receiving a massage therapy using essential oils

✓ By soaking in an oil-infused bath

As you continue reading this book, you will understand the various kinds of essential oils and how you can use them to achieve the best results for your body and well-being.

Chapter 2: Health and Healing

Benefits of Essential Oils

Physical Health

Essential oils have been proven to support physical well-being time and time again. They can be used as part of a concoction or separately. Thousands of communities and millions of people across the world have used (and continue to use) the following essences and essential oils to help treat or reduce inflammation for certain physical ailments. Here are some of the most well-known and the physical ailments they can assist with:

> Angelica Root Oil - Psoriasis, Dull skin, Water retention by the body, Gout and Toxin build up
>
> Anise Oil - Flu, Bronchitis, Muscle aches, Rheumatism, Flatulence and Coughs
>
> Basil Oil - Sinusitis, Gout, Bronchitis, Muscle aches, Insect bites, Rheumatism, Exhaustion, Flu and Coughs
>
> Bay Leaf Oil - Poor circulation, hair Care, Neuralgia, Dandruff, Sprains and Oily Skin

Bay Laurel - Flu, Tonsillitis, Colds, Loss of appetite and Amenorrhea

Benzoin Oil - Chapped skin, Laryngitis, Amenorrhea, Flu and Colds

Bergamot Oil - Oily skin, Psoriasis, Acne, Boils, Cold sores and Halitosis

Bois de Rose (Rosewood Oil) - Oily skin, Scars, Acne, Colds, Sensitive skin, Stretch marks, Fever and Flu

Cajeput Oil - Sore throat, Muscle aches, Oily skin, Rheumatism, Sinusitis, Asthma and Bronchitis

Cardamom Oil - Halitosis, Loss of appetite and Coli

Carrot Seed Oil - Gout, Toxin build up and Eczema

Cedar Wood Atlas Oil - Dermatitis, Dandruff, Arthritis, Coughing, Bronchitis and Acne

Cedar Wood Oil - Dermatitis, Dandruff, Arthritis, Coughing, Bronchitis and Acne

German Chamomile Essence - Sores, Sprains, Rheumatism, Allergies, Colic Cuts, Hair care, Headaches, PMS, Strains, Dermatitis,

Inflamed skin, Flatulence, Abscesses and Neuralgia

Roman Chamomile Essence - Sores, Sprains, Rheumatism, Allergies, Colic Cuts, Hair care, Headaches, PMS, Strains, Dermatitis, Inflamed skin, Flatulence, Abscesses and Neuralgia

Cinnamon Oil - Scabies, Flatulence, Constipation, Lice, Low blood pressure and Exhaustion

Citronella Essence - Oily skin, Fatigue, Headache, Excessive perspiration and Insect bites

Clary Sage Oil - Sore throat, Asthma, Amenorrhea, Labor pains and Coughing

Clove Bud Oil - Asthma, Sprains, Arthritis, Toothache, and Rheumatism

Coriander Oil - Nausea, Gout, Colic, Aches, Indigestion and Rheumatism

Cypress Oil - Hemorrhoids, Oily Skin, Excessive perspiration and Varicose veins

Elemi Oil - Wounds, Scars, Bronchitis, Coughing and Catarrh

Eucalyptus Globulous Oil - Sinusitis, Arthritis, Cold sores, Poor circulation, Flu and Fever

Fennel Oil - Toxin build up, Flatulence, Halitosis, Nausea and Cellulite

Frankincense - Stretch marks, Bronchitis, Coughing, Scars and Asthma

Galbanum Oil - Scars, Muscle aches, Bronchitis, Cuts, Sores, Lice, Acne and Boils

Geranium Oil - Lice, Oily skin, Acne and Cellulite

Ginger Oil - Nausea, Muscle ache, Arthritis and Poor circulation

Grapefruit Oil - Toxin build up, Cellulite and Dull skin

Helichrysum Oil - Boils, Wounds, Cuts, Acne, Burns, Abscesses and Eczema

Hyssop Oil - Sore throat, Bruises and Coughing

Jasmine Oil - Sensitive skin, Dry skin and Labor pains

Juniper Berry Oil - Gout, Toxin build up, Cellulite, Rheumatism and Hemorrhoids

Lavender Oil - Oily skin, Itchy skin, Headache, Cuts, Stretch marks, Acne, Flatulence, Allergies, Asthma, Insect bites, Insect repellant, Sprains, Colic Burns, Scabies and Scars

Lemon Oil - Oily skin, Varicose veins, Colds, Athlete's foot and Warts

Lemongrass Oil - Oily skin, Acne, Scabies, Athlete's foot, Excessive perspiration and Flatulence

Linden Blossom Oil - Scars, Spots, Oily skin, Headaches, Migraines and Wrinkles

Marjoram Oil - Sprains, Cramps, Muscle ache, Arthritis, Migraine and Neuralgia

Melissa Oil - Herpes, Shingles, Cold sores, Flu and Indigestion

Myrrh - Halitosis, Athlete's foot, Bronchitis, Ringworm and Amenorrhea

Myrtle - Coughs, Irritated skin and Asthma

Neroli - Stretch marks, Scars and Oily skin

Niaouli - Colds, Coughs, Sore throat, Bronchitis, Acne and Oily skin

Nutmeg Oil - Muscle ache, Constipation, Poor circulation, Nausea and Rheumatism

Bitter Orange Oil - Flatulence, Flu, Colds, Constipation, Dull skin and Bleeding gums

Oregano Oil - Respiration, Colds and Digestion

Parsley Oil - Kidney complications, Digestion, Congestion and Diuretic

Patchouli Oil - Oily skin, Dandruff, Eczema, Acne, Chapped skin, Dermatitis and Cellulite

Black Pepper Oil - Constipation, Detox, Muscle ache, Muscle cramps, Poor circulation and Arthritis

Peppermint Oil - Vertigo, Exhaustion, Fever, Flatulence, Nausea, Asthma, Scabies and Sinusitis

Petit-grain Oil - Insomnia and Rapid heartbeat

Pine Oil - Flu, Sinusitis, Colds and Congestion

Rose Oil - Eczema

Rosemary Oil - Muscle ache, Hair care, Gout, Neuralgia, Arthritis, rheumatism, Dandruff and Exhaustion

Sandalwood Oil - Urinary tract problems, Bronchitis, Oily skin and Strep throat

Spearmint Oil - Nausea, Headache, Asthma, Exhaustion, Scabies and Flatulence

Thyme Oil - Dermatitis, Arthritis, Bronchitis, Cuts and Laryngitis

Vetiver Oil - Oily skin, Muscle aches, Arthritis and Rheumatism

Violet Leaf Oil - Insomnia, Bronchitis, Poor circulation and Congestion

Yarrow Oil - Hypertension, Inflammation, Arthritis, Acne, Hair care and Insomnia

Ylang Ylang Oil - Palpitations, Hypertension and PMS symptoms

Essential oils are also beneficial emotionally and mentally. Below I've noted benefits of various oils when it comes to reducing or resolving a number of emotional issues.

Angelica Root Oil - Stress and Nervousness

Anise Oil - Depression

Basil Oil - Exhaustion, Burnout and Fatigue

Bay Leaf Oil - Emotional exhaustion

Bay Laurel - Confidence booster

Benzoin Oil - Emotional insecurities

Bergamot Oil - Emotional insecurities, Anger, Anxiety, Depression, Fatigue and Confidence

Bois de Rose (Rosewood Oil) - Emotional imbalance and Depression

Cajeput Oil - Mental Fatigue and Emotional Confusion

Cardamom Oil - Guilt feelings, Stress and Shame

Carrot Seed Oil - Mood swings, Mental exhaustion, Stress and Anxiety

Cedar Wood Atlas Oil - Anxieties, Insecurities and Stress

Cedar Wood Oil - Anxieties, Insecurities and Stress

German Chamomile Essence - Anxieties, Insecurities, Depression, Loneliness and Stress

Roman Chamomile Essence - Irritability, Anxiety, Emotional Stress, Depression, Fear and Insomnia

Cinnamon Oil - Mental Concentration and Emotional and Mental Fatigue

Citronella Essence - Mind fog and Tension

Clary Sage Oil - Loneliness, Mental stress and Fear

Clove Bud Oil - Mental concentration and Depression

Coriander Oil - Irritability and Fatigue

Cypress Oil - Grief, Confidence issues and Mental concentration

Elemi Oil - Grief and Agitation

Eucalyptus Globulous Oil - Mental concentration

Fennel Oil - Emotional imbalance

Frankincense - Depression, Panic attacks, Anxiety, Loneliness, Grief, Emotional insecurities and Mental exhaustion

Galbanum Oil - Nervousness, Mood swings and Emotional rigidity

Geranium Oil - Anxiety, Emotional imbalance, Depression and Stress

Ginger Oil - Mental exhaustion and Burnout

Grapefruit Oil - Confidence issues, Stress, Fear and Depression

Helichrysum Oil - Loneliness, Grief and Panic Attacks

Hyssop Oil - Mental concentration and Nervousness

Jasmine Oil - Depression, Emotional fatigue, Stress, Confidence issues and Burnout

Juniper Berry Oil - Negative energy and Agitation

Lavender Oil - Panic attacks, Anxiety and Irritability

Lemon Oil - Memory issues and Fear

Lemongrass Oil - Emotional and mental confusion

Linden Blossom Oil - Stress and Tension

Marjoram Oil - Mood swings and PMS symptoms

Melissa Oil - Nervousness, Tension and Agitation

Myrrh - Emotional imbalance and Creativity

Myrtle - Depression, Addiction and Self-destructive tendencies

Neroli - Irritability, Anxiety, Stress and Panic attacks

Niaouli - Emotional concentration

Nutmeg Oil - Mental fatigue

Bitter Orange Oil - Depression, Confidence issues and Stress

Oregano Oil - Emotional insecurities

Parsley Oil - Emotional and mental rigidity

Patchouli Oil - Mental and emotional exhaustion and Stress

Black Pepper Oil - Emotional and mental fatigue and Anxiety

Peppermint Oil - Burnout, Mental concentration and Emotional fatigue

Petit-grain Oil - Panic attacks and Anxiety

Pine Oil - Depression, Nervousness and Exhaustion

Rose Oil - Panic attacks, Depression, Grief, Loneliness and Stress

Rosemary Oil - Mental exhaustion, Confidence issues, Burnout and Mental concentration

Sandalwood Oil - Stress, Irritability, Anxiety and Depression

Spearmint Oil - Depression and Mental and Emotional fatigue

Thyme Oil - Mental concentration

Vetiver Oil - Anger, Emotional insecurities, Grief and Stress

Violet Leaf Oil - Nostalgia obsession and Shyness

Yarrow Oil - Tension, Stress and Insomnia

Ylang Ylang Oil - Mood swings, Stress and Anger

Spiritual Health

Human beings have also incorporated essential oils and essences in prayers and spiritual journeys. Some of the oldest accounts of these have been recorded in The Bible and Holy Quran as well as historical accounts dating back to the Egyptian Empire and Ancient Indians which we explored in Chapter 1 of this book. Spiritual journeys are personal and vary from individual to individual and different essential oils speak out uniquely to different people. However, through extensive research, I was able to find that essential oils help in the following areas:

- ✓ Purification of the soul
- ✓ Promoting a harmonious environment
- ✓ Promoting love for one another
- ✓ Offering meaningful prayers while connecting to your higher power
- ✓ Harnessing the virtue of patience

Household Uses of Essential Oils

With seemingly endless choices of essential oils and their uses, often times, people get confused and overwhelmed as to what exactly to buy and how to use it. Now, around the house and for day to day activities, essential oils can work miracles. Here's how you can put your essential oil collection to work for your household purposes.

- ✓ You can deodorize the air around your house and in your fridge with lime oil and grapefruit oil.
- ✓ Get rid of that persistent pungent smell from your trash bin with geranium or lemon oil sprinkled into baking soda.

- ✓ Wipe dusty surfaces clean and stain by using orange oil, lemon oil or grapefruit oil.
- ✓ Make an insect repellant out of your peppermint oil, lavender oil, lemongrass oil, and citronella or rosemary oil.
- ✓ Clean your kids' sports outfit by adding tea tree oil and lemon oil to baking soda and warm water.
- ✓ Whip up peppermint patties for guests by using coconut oil, peppermint oil, dark chocolate and raw honey.
- ✓ Give scents to your washed clothes by adding a few drops of your favorite essence to the load in your washing machine.
- ✓ Make a DIY carpet cleaner powder by adding some tea tree oil to Borax.
- ✓ You can also use lemon oil mixed with water to wash fresh fruits and vegetables.
- ✓ Keep your shoes' odor at bay by infusing lemon oil, geranium oil, basil oil or lavender oil.
- ✓ Neutralize pet odor with a proper mixture of lavender oil or geranium with vinegar.

✓ Get rid of mites from your beddings by washing them with Eucalyptus oil mixed with water.

✓ Whip up a bunch of quick homemade recipes such as: mint tea and flavored lemon water, using your favorite essential oils.

Household uses of essential oil are practically limitless. Putting these oils to proper use will give you and your family the much needed calmness, comfort and tranquility living in a clean and peaceful environment.

Busting 5 Most Common Essential Oils Myths

Worldwide awareness of the fantastic healing properties of essential oils will continue to grow, but it is important that we dispel the misinformation about what these healing compounds are and what they can do. Much of the misinformation and myths involving essential oils are rooted in personal desire or corporate desire to sell more oils to unsuspecting people. So, let's set the record straight on some of the myths about essential oils.

Myth #1: Essential Oils Cures Everything for Everyone

In our collective effort to heal the world naturally, we must be careful not to get caught up in the one-size-fits-all fallacy. The success you may discover with one type of oil may not have the same result for your friend. We often see fallacious conclusions to explain this discrepancy with the following statements:

"You didn't pray hard enough or believe well enough"

"You must have received the bad batch of the oil"

"You didn't use this oil correctly"

"Essential oils simply don't work"

Our bodies respond differently to the complex compounds of essential oil. Where you find success with one type of essential oil, your friend might find the same success for the same condition with a completely different type of essential oil. Seek out every natural option to improve your health but be open to the fact that essential oils might not be the end-all fix for the condition you are targeting.

Myth #2: Essential Oils Labeled as "Therapeutic Grade" or "Clinical Grade" are of the Highest Quality

There is no governing body that certifies grades of essential oil. The quality behind an essential oil has more to its story that can be revealed by a GC-MS test (Grade Chromatography-Mass Spectrometry). Therapeutic Grade and Clinical Grade are great examples but not an exhaustive list of marketing terms made up by certain companies to set their oils above that of the other companies. The companies producing the oil decides to label their oils with these terms; not a third party authority. As an individual user, you should be interested in what the company's position is on the quality of the oils they are selling.

Therefore, you should make plans to do a little more research and ask a few more questions about how the company produces their essential oils to get a clearer picture of the quality rather than shopping for oil simply based on a company's chosen marketing term.

Myth #3: The Best Place to Apply Essential Oils are the Soles of the Feet

Massage Today and Aromatherapy United debunked this popular practice. Dermatology science shows that our stratum corneum (the outermost layer of skin) is the thickest on the soles of our feet which makes it more difficult for essential oils to penetrate cell membranes. While it is true that our feet are very porous when compared to the rest of our body, it is also true that these pores are mostly sweat glands that are not a reliable delivery method to the blood. Alternatively, the stratum corneum on the arms, back, legs and abdomen are much thinner and much more effective locations for penetration of essential oils.

Myth #4: With Essential Oils, You Always Get What You Pay For

This phrase is commonly used by companies or individuals selling higher price oils. While it can be true that you get what you pay for, it is also true that you can overpay for what you get. If you are willing to pay a higher price for a brand that others can't afford or you simply aren't willing to overpay, it is important to understand that higher priced oil is not always an indication that the oil is of higher quality. Price considerations should certainly be part of your evaluation process when deciding what brands of oil you would like to purchase. However, don't fall victim to the misconception that the price of the oil automatically makes that oil higher-quality.

Myth #5: Best Quality Essential Oils Never Deteriorate or Expire

If it were possible to store essential oils in a completely oxygen-free atmosphere, then there could possibly be some truth to this myth. However, in the world we live in, everything oxidizes and breaks down with time – even 100% pure essential oils. Nonetheless, proper care of your essential oil bottles will allow your oils to last for years. This should include storing your oils in a dark, cool place away from direct sunlight and keeping your lids tight when not in use.

Chapter 3: A Word for Beginners

Essential Oil Safety Tips for Beginners

Keep Out of Eyes, Ears and Open Wounds (Burns, Cuts and Bruises)

Avoid getting oil in your eyes or ears. You'll want to avoid contact with any sensitive areas or wounds on the body; so make sure you wash your hands after applying the oils. If you happen to get a little oil in your eyes, flush it out with olive, vegetable or fractionated coconut oil. To flush your eyes with oil you can use a tissue and gently wipe the area. Your natural reaction might be to use water; however, keep in mind that oil and water don't mix. Using water might actually make things worse.

Always Read the Label

Be sure to look at the oil's label and review the provided product guide for usage and directions. Many oils can be used internally, topically and aromatically; however, not all of the oils can be used with all three application methods. You'll also want to note the provided sensitivity chart and make sure you are diluting the oil properly. If you have sensitive skin, you might want to keep some carrier oil handy when trying the oil for the first time.

Avoid Topical Usage of Citrus Oils in Direct Sunlight

Avoid using citrus oils topically when going into direct sunlight. This is because citrus oils can be photosensitive and can cause discoloration of the skin. Even using a tanning bed and using the citrus oils topically should be avoided.

Internal Consumption

Not all essential oils can be consumed internally. Typically, oils safe for internal consumption will be labeled by the FDA as GRAS (generally recognized as safe). Also, they will ordinarily come with a supplement facts box with dietary supplement, warnings and instructions.

Usage when Pregnant

It is advisable that you consult your doctor before using any essential oil when pregnant or under a doctor's care. Depending on your health condition, your physician will be able to properly advise you on what essential oils you can use and how to use them.

Remember that because essential oils are quite potent, a little goes a long way. You only need a few drops to experience the incredible benefits that come with their usage.

Ways to Use Essential Oils

As you already know by now, uses of essential oils are endless. Application of these oils can be done in a number of ways which vary based on the type of oil, the purpose for which it is being used as well as the effects of the oil on human skin. Without further ado, let us consider the following types of applications.

Skin Application

Due to their fat soluble nature, essential oils are almost immediately absorbed by the skin when applied. However, most people like to mix and dilute them with a neutral carrier oil such as coconut oil or sweet almond oil. More about carrier oils will be addressed in the next sub-topic. A common concern when using carrier oils is that they tend to go rancid therefore choice of carrier oils, for most people, is based on its smell, texture and sensitivities. The wrists, feet, behind the ears and temples are the most popular areas of application.

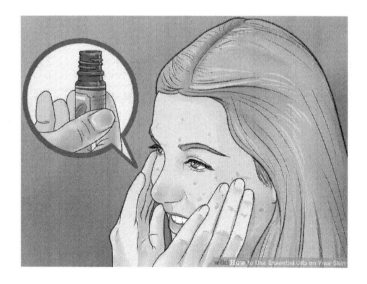

Simple Inhalation

This method involves pouring a few drops of your favorite oil onto the palm of your hands, rubbing them gently and briefly and then inhaling. Alternatively, you can pour a few drops on a tissue and inhale. For beginners, a couple of drops are enough to avoid any reactions or sensitivities.

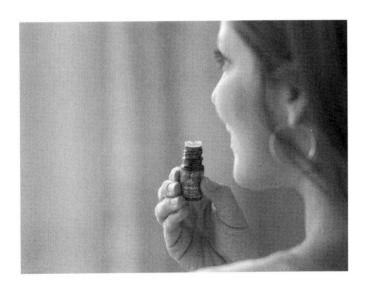

Steam Inhalation

For steam inhalation, boil about 3 cups of water, pour into a bowl and add a few drops of your favorite oil. Now, place your nose about 10 inches from the bowl, cover your head with a cloth or towel and gently inhale the steam. You'd be surprised how relaxing this can become.

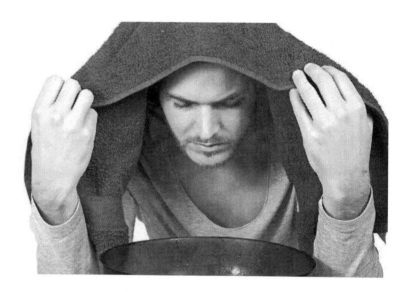

There are different types of electronic diffusers. They are convenient because all you have to do is feed a few drops of your favorite oil into the diffuser, turn it on and circulate in your room. Electronic diffusers are pretty simple to use and maintain.

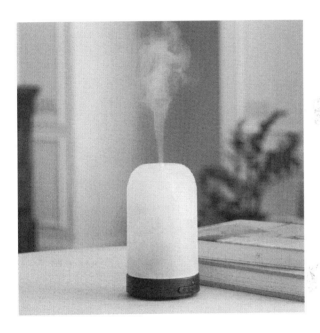

Application through Baths

One of the most relaxing ways to unwind after a long or busy day is by soaking your body in a bath. Essential oils take this experience to a whole new level. Normally, you would use salts, such as Epsom salt, as the base to ensure that the oil you are adding dissolves properly for the best results. Remember not to use any chemically produced soap(s) during this relaxing bath time.

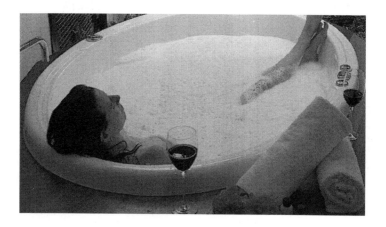

For aromatherapy massage purposes, essential oils are mixed with neutral-smelling carrier oils such as grape seed oil or sweet almond oil. Measurements vary but anything in the neighborhood of a ratio of 20 drops of essential oil to an ounce of carrier oil should work just fine.

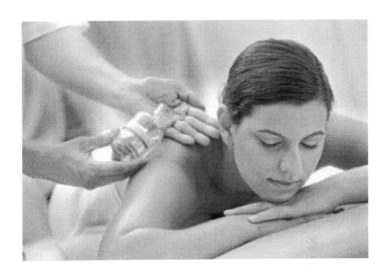

Carrier Oils

Carrier oils are a naturally derived vegetable oil of neutral smell. They are obtained from the fatty portion of a plant. Unlike essential oils, carrier oils are not volatile; making them perfect as a dilution medium. In a way, you could describe carrier oils as the indispensable companion of topically applied essential oils. Some of the most common types of carrier oils include:

- Coconut oil
- Olive oil
- Sweet almond oil
- Grapeseed oil
- Castor oil
- Flaxseed oil
- Jojoba oil
- Avocado oil
- Apricot kernel oil
- Black seed oil

Because they are high in fat, carrier oils have a limited shelf life which varies from six months to one year. To get maximum shelf life, carrier oils should be stored in an air tight container and in a dark cool place.

You can use carrier oils to make your own blends. If you have smaller vials, you can add some carrier oil to it along with a mixture of your essential oils to make your own custom blends. Carrier oils can also be used as massage oils by adding about 15 to 25 drops of essential oil to an ounce of carrier oil such as coconut oil.

Carrier oils come in handy if you accidentally apply essential oil in a sensitive part of your skin or body such as the eyes; since washing it out with water will make things worse.

Buying Your First Essential Oils

Best 5 Essential Oils to Buy Under $100

There are tons of essential oils out there with numerous applications as well as varying price ranges. As a beginner, the information alone can get quite overwhelming. There is no doubt that essential oils have benefits, but that does not mean that every dealer or supplier of these products sell them at fair market price. Granted, there's a lot that goes into determining prices for different oils. Factors like the cost of distillation and availability of the parent plant, among others, play a key role in setting the price. That said, for beginners looking to buy good essential oils under $100, the following should be easily available:

- ✓ Lavender Oil
- ✓ Peppermint Oil
- ✓ Lemon Oil
- ✓ Frankincense

Finding a Good Supplier

It is no secret that essential oils continue to rise in popularity. They are much more readily available than they were, say, three decades ago. Many brands are popping up every year which also comes with an increase in unscrupulous suppliers. So, how do you maneuver this market without getting swindled? Well, before choosing any supplier, take into account the following:

Consider the Supplier's Pricing of Essential Oils

If the price looks too good to be true, it probably is. A lot of factors affect the final price of essential oils. The distillation process of extracting the oil is quite expensive as it is. Add to that the availability of the base plant and the physical and chemical properties of the oil and you can begin to understand why oils are priced differently. For example, at least 260 pounds of rose blossoms are needed to produce an ounce of rose oil. This should tell you that rose oil can't be cheap. A little research into a product you are interested in can go a long way in helping you decide whether you purchase it from supplier X or supplier Y.

Research on the Products' Purity and Testing

Since there is no standardized test for essential oil carried out by an independent third party, the issue of purity often gets a little tricky. As a general rule, make a point of finding out what purity tests the suppliers' brands perform and how they do it. Purity can be affected by seasons as well as where the plants grow.

A brand that explains to its customers, in detail, the extensive tests they carry out on their products and provide some sort of evidence for this builds a lot more trust. Also, as an essential oil user, you should check out reviews by past users of the same brand to help you make a decision.

Chapter 4: Essential Oils and Their Uses

The Top 50 Essential Oils

As you already know, essential oils come from plants. Every plant has its own unique aroma and therapeutic benefits, so it is only logical that the number of essential oils be in the hundreds, if not thousands. Naturally, this presents a challenge to many people when it comes to choosing essential oils to address different concerns. I did extensive research in the various essential oils available out there and came up with a shortlist of the top 53 most popular essential oils based on their multifold uses, availability, affordability and effectiveness. You should know that the following is just a list of the essential oils. The next chapter will discuss them in much more detail with respect to their multiple uses.

Basil Oil	Bergamot Oil	Cardamom Oil
Carrot Seed Oil	Cassia Oil	Cedar Wood Oil
Cilantro Oil	Cinnamon Oil	Clary Sage Oil
Clove Oil	Cypress Oil	Eucalyptus Oil
Fennel Oil	Frankincense Oil	Geranium Oil

German Chamomile Oil	Ginger Oil	Grapefruit Oil
Helichrysum Oil	Jasmine Oil	Jojoba Oil
Juniper Oil	Lavender Oil	Lemon Oil
Lemongrass Oil	Lime Oil	Marjoram Oil
Melaleuca Oil	Myrrh Oil	Neroli Oil
Oregano Oil	Palmarosa Oil	Patchouli Oil
Peppermint Oil	Pine Oil	Pomegranate Seed Oil
Roman Chamomile Oil	Rose Oil	Rosehip Oil
Rosemary Oil Sweet	Sandalwood Oil	Orange Oil
Tangerine Oil	Tarragon Oil	Tea Tree Oil
Thyme Oil	Turmeric Oil	Vetiver Oil
White Fir Oil	Wild Orange Oil	Wintergreen Oil
Yarrow Oil	Ylang-Ylang Oil	

Chapter 5: Best 3 in 10 Categories

Top 3 Essential Oils for Energy and Vitality

Peppermint Essential Oil

Peppermint essential oil has many uses, especially in terms of its shear medicinal value. Its active ingredient is menthol, which is found in high concentrations. This makes peppermint essential oil one of the strongest natural antibacterial, anti-fungal and anti-viral oils. Its strong, invigorating, minty aroma makes it excellent for boosting both mental and physical vitality. It has been used to boost concentration, fight fatigue and improve exercise performance.

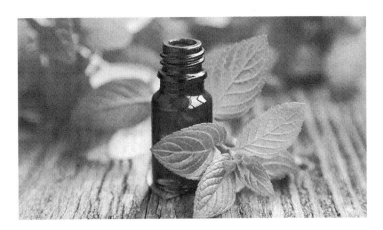

There are three ways in which you can use peppermint essential oil to boost energy and vitality. They are as follows:

- Combine 1 drop of peppermint oil and 1 drop rosehip oil; rub them together and gently apply under your nose, base of your neck or shoulders.
- Add some to your diffuser and turn it on when you are studying or working on a project. It will help you concentrate and stay alert.
- You can also just inhale it directly. Ideally, you would do this before your workouts to help prevent lethargy while also giving you the energy and drive you need.

Eucalyptus Essential Oil

The main compound found in eucalyptus oil is cineole. It is a powerhouse of healing properties and has been found to feature antioxidant, anti-inflammatory and analgesic properties. Thanks to its multipurpose nature, many researchers have been drawn to study it. Findings from a 2010 study led to eucalyptus oil being described as an "immune-stimulator" with the capabilities of boosting energy levels in the body.

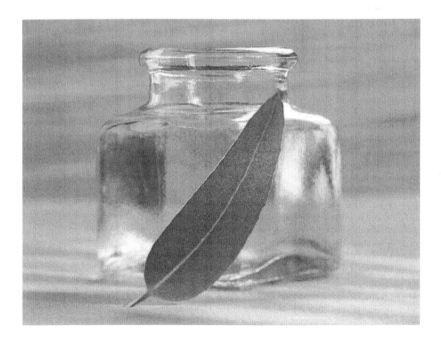

How to Use Eucalyptus Essential Oil

- Apply topically by rubbing a few drops of the oil on your wrists, muscles and temple after a long day. The tingling effect has a surprisingly strong calming effect.
- Add a few drops to your diffuser and let the menthol molecules provide an energizing aromatherapy.
- Add some drops to your shower to relieve the fatigue that comes with a cold. It will also uplift your mood.
- Direct inhalation from the bottle will provide you with an instant energy wake-me-up.

When you are short on sleep and looking for something to jumpstart your mojo, ginger essential oil is your buddy. This spicy oil is great for maintaining energy levels, fighting feelings of sluggishness and revitalization.

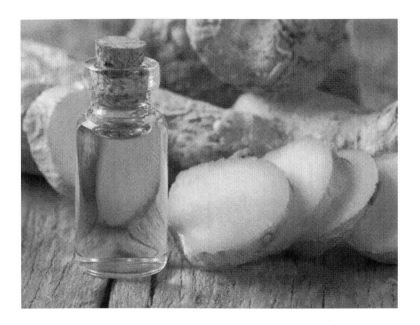

How to Use Ginger Essential Oil

- You can inhale it directly from the bottle. Its hot aroma not only elevates your energy levels, it also fights off feelings of nausea or morning sickness – whether you are hungover or pregnant. For those interested in weight loss or maintaining a diet, this oil is known to reduce cravings and appetite.

- For topical application, add about 3 drops of ginger oil to some carrier oil such as Moringa oil and rub on your hands and feet. Once it is absorbed into the bloodstream, your vitality increases, senses become stimulated and overall energy is boosted.

Top 3 Essential Oils for Anxiety and Mental Health

Lavender Essential Oil

Lavender essential oil has a very fresh and floral aroma which is quite calming and relaxing. Referred to as an "adapt-o-gen", lavender essential oil is one of the most ideal picks for enhancing mood. Its nature as a mood enhancer makes it good for reducing stress, insomnia and calming agitation. There is growing scientific evidence that suggests topical application of anxiety-relieving essential oils is the most effective. Lavender oil has been found to enter the bloodstream within just a few minutes of rubbing on the skin.

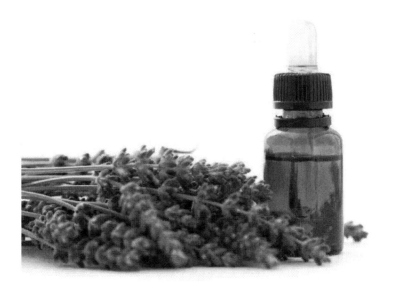

How to Use Lavender Essential Oil

- Rub a few drops onto your palm and inhale directly. The oil penetrates to the center of emotions – also known as the amygdala – providing instant relaxation. Use it in high-stress areas such very crowded areas or in the office.

- Rub a few drops into your temples to ease tension and relieve headaches.

- Add a couple of drops in hot water to make a lavender herbal tea. It is very soothing and relaxing.

Cedar Wood Essential Oil

Cedar wood oil is yet another essential oil known for its stress relieving and calming properties. Once it penetrates the bloodstream, the aroma triggers the release of serotonin – a chemical that stabilizes mood in the brain. Serotonin can also be converted to melatonin to promote calmness and regulate sleep patterns; so, in effect, cedar wood essential oil is also a natural sedative.

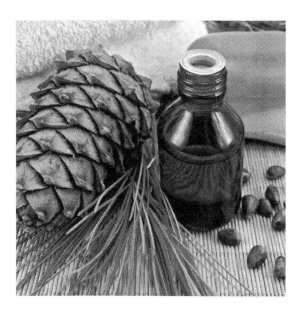

- You can either rub a few drops on a handkerchief or the palm of your hands and inhale; or just inhale directly from the bottle.
- Rub some drops onto your neck or above your eyebrows to relieve tension.
- You can also, add some to your diffuser and let it waft through the air covering the whole room.

Grapefruit Essential Oil

Grapefruit essential oil is another type of citrus-based oil whose aroma is refreshing, uplifting and clarifying. The fruit itself has almost similar effects to lime. This stress-buster oil alleviates depression, mental fatigue and headaches resulting from stress. A simple whiff can go a long way in transforming your whole day for the better.

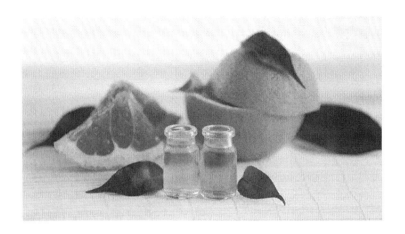

How to Use Grapefruit Essential Oil

- Using a diffuser to diffuse grapefruit oil aroma is perhaps the best way to tap into its effectiveness. Add a few drops in your diffuser and let it fill your room with anxiety-relieving aroma.

- You can also apply it topically. Along with some carrier oil such as jojoba or grapeseed oil, add a few drops to a cotton pad and gently rub onto your wrists and neck.

- Add some drops to your shower and cover the drain. As the water falls on your body, inhale deeply to enjoy its anxiety-relieving benefits.

Top 3 Essential Oils for Haircare

Rosemary Essential Oil

Rosemary essential oil is another multipurpose oil whose powerful effects are only matched by its fresh minty and woodsy scent; as Up Nature puts it: *"Rosemary's aroma is instantly youthful and deliciously herbaceous"*.

When it comes to haircare, rosemary oil is one of the most popular essential oils. It has a lot of antioxidants which stimulate hair follicles and prevent graying and thinning of hair. If you are struggling with an itchy scalp, rosemary oil can provide a great relief for dandruff while clearing pores. It also tones down the production of sebum which helps a lot with oily scalps.

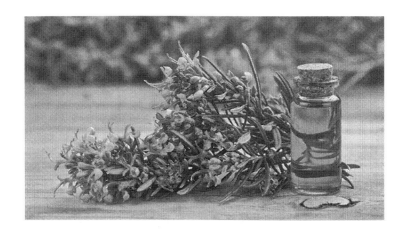

How to Use Rosemary Essential Oil for Haircare

Heat about 3 to 4 tablespoons of olive oil over medium heat and blend in about a dozen drops of rosemary essential oil a few minutes later. Once thoroughly mixed, pour this oil treatment over your head and rub into your scalp. Dip a towel in hot water and wrap your hair with it and leave it for half an hour before shampooing it out. Make a point of doing this once a month and your hair will transform for the better.

Clary Sage Essential Oil

Of all sages, the clary sage is probably the most versatile. It has a distinct murky aroma; however, what makes it a good fit for hair care is its phytoestrogen content that is known to prevent, and in some cases reverse, premature balding. If you are suffering from excess dandruff production, clary sage oil can help to normalize your scalp's production of oil. It is not ideal for use when you are pregnant since it is known to induce contractions.

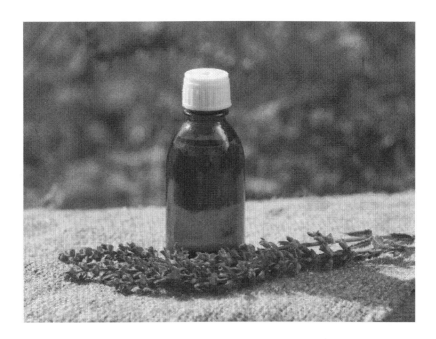

If you intend to use clary sage oil to promote hair growth, blend equal parts of the oil and jojoba oil then rub it into your scalp. Give it about half an hour before shampooing it out.

Patchouli Essential Oil

Because patchouli has a very strong aroma, it is recommended that you use it in small amounts. This deep, earthy and sensual oil has antiseptic and anti-inflammatory properties which make it ideal for treating skin irritations. With patchouli essential oil, dandruff and eczema can quickly become a thing of the past. Hair loss brought by eczema can also be resolved in the process.

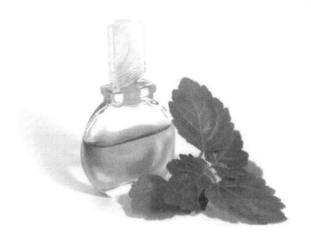

How to Use Patchouli Essential Oils

Blend together 1 part patchouli oil, 2 parts rosemary oil and 3 parts argan oil. Take this blend and massage it generously and deeply into your scalp and leave it for a couple of hours before shampooing it out.

Top 3 Essential Oils for Skincare, Aging and Acne

Frankincense Essential Oil

Frankincense essential oil promotes skin cell regeneration, meaning it prevents aging of the skin, making users look much more youthful. It also heals scars while reducing the appearance of wrinkles and lines.

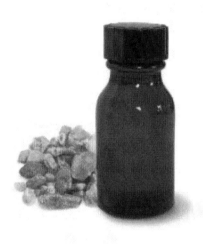

How to Use Frankincense Essential Oils

Using this oil before you go to sleep at night helps the skin rejuvenate much faster while you sleep. Take a couple of drops of frankincense and blend it together with almond oil then apply it to your already cleansed and moisturized face. This blend can serve as a night mask. In case you made more than enough, you can store the excess blend in a dark glass container for future use.

Geranium Essential Oil

Geranium essential oil contains a lot of antioxidants which help fight signs of aging. The antioxidants work by fighting off the free radicals that your skin is exposed to on a daily basis. Thanks to its astringent properties, geranium oil can normalize oil production of the skin. This makes it an ideal choice for people struggling with oily skin. It makes the skin look more youthful by reducing the appearance of large, open pores.

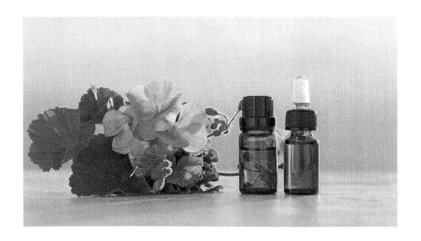

How to Use Geranium Essential Oil

Geranium controls excess oil and breakouts thereby giving life to your skin. You can use it as a moisturizer. An ideal blend can be made mixing 1 part geranium oil with 5 parts jojoba oil that you apply as a primer before using your makeup.

Carrot Seed Essential Oil

Carrot seed oil reverses the harsh effects that occur on your skin when it is exposed to unhealthy environmental conditions over a long period of time. Before you leave the house, apply a few drops of this oil mixed with your favorite carrier oil. It helps maintain the youthful glow of your skin for longer periods of time.

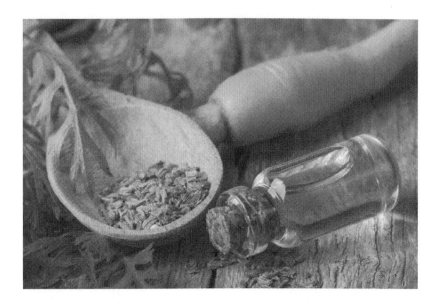

How to Use Carrot Seed Essential Oil

Mix a few drops of carrot seed oil with some carrier oil such as jojoba oil and apply it to your skin. If you have oily skin, make a toner by adding some drops of carrot seed oil and apricot kernel oil to some rosewater and spray it on your face before applying your moisturizer.

Top 3 Essential Oils for Sleep and Relaxation

Roman Chamomile Essential Oil

Chamomile, in general, is quite popular for fighting insomnia; however, the Roman Chamomile is perhaps the strongest of all of them. Chamomile is an ancient herb that has therapeutic properties that relax the body and mind, hence acting as a sedative. So it comes as no surprise that it is a common pick for treating stress and nervous tension as well. In addition, its sweet and comforting scent has been found to treat hysteria and insomnia.

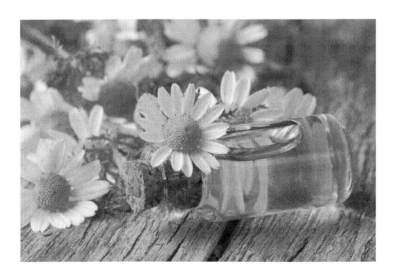

- Add a few drops to the palm of your hands or a handkerchief and inhale deeply. You can also just inhale directly from the bottle.
- Add about 2 drops to a cup of black tea for that soothing feeling before you go to bed.

Bergamot Essential Oil

Bergamot essential oil is citrus-based and has one of the most pleasant smells of all essential oils. Recent studies have now confirmed what was believed that this oil greatly reduces anxiety and improves mood. What it does is cuts down the amount of cortisol in the saliva, giving it some sedative properties. By doing this, you get to spend more time in the restorative stage of sleep.

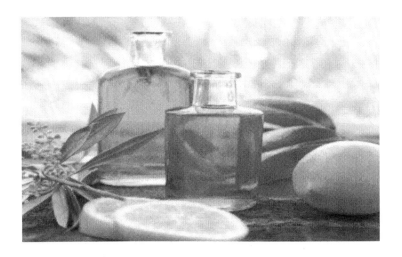

How to Use Bergamot Essential Oil

- Take a few drops of this oil, rub on the palm of your hands then cover your nose with your hands as you inhale deeply.
- For topical application, rub some of this oil on the back of your neck or temples before going to bed.

Lavender Essential Oil

There is no doubt that lavender oil is a powerhouse when it comes to multi-fold uses. It consistently features among the top and most popular choices of essential oils for various uses. It is made up of esters and alcohols that have therapeutic properties, such as relaxation. True lavender essential oil reigns supreme over other forms of lavender oil such as spike lavender and lavandin oils. It calms nerves, reduces the effects of asthma, improves digestion and relieves headaches; laying all the groundwork for a good night's sleep.

How to Use Lavender Essential Oil

- Rub a few drops onto your palm and inhale directly. The oil penetrates to the center of emotions – also known as the amygdala – providing instant relaxation. Use it in high-stress areas such very crowded areas or in the office.
- Rub a few drops into your temples to ease tension and relieve headaches.
- Add a couple of drops in hot water to make a lavender herbal tea. It is very soothing and relaxing.

Top 3 Essential Oils for Happiness and Mood

Ylang Ylang Essential Oil

The flower of this oil have an incredibly sweet and floral aroma that reduces the negative thoughts associated with depression and mood swings. Ylang ylang has already been seeing usage in mainstream and high-end perfume brands like Chanel. A recent study described this oil as, *"a relief for depression and stress in humans"*. It reduces stress levels, uplifts spirits and promotes happiness and calmness.

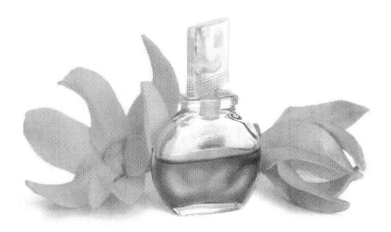

- Apply topically by rubbing a few drops on your neck, wrists, and feet or behind your ears.

Sandalwood Essential Oil

Sandalwood is often found in incense. It has a woody, warm and calming aroma which helps clear your mind and help with meditation. The oil's scent is regarded as a strong emotional balancer thanks to its effect on the brain's limbic system. Not only does it enhance sleep quality through its sedative properties, it also reduces the feelings of depression.

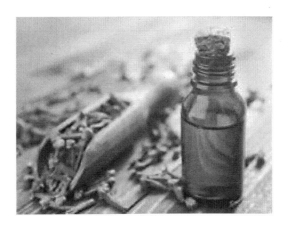

- You can inhale directly from its bottle or rub some onto the palm of your hands and inhaling.
- Add about 6 drops of this oil to 2 drops of rose oil and blend with jojoba oil then use this new blend to massage your wrists, feet and back.

Basil Essential Oil

Basil oil is very high in vitamin C and antioxidants which are known to calm the nerves and reduce inflammation. While Depression and happiness are polar opposites, Basil is known to help with both. Basil oil revitalizes energy levels, alleviates chronic fatigue and promotes calmness; all of which work against depression. This lays the foundation for a good mood (and happiness along the way).

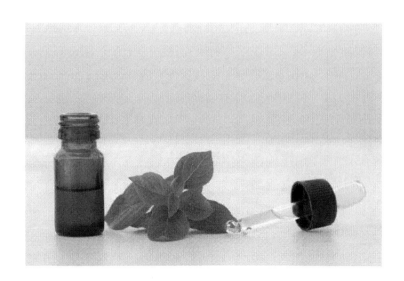

How to Use Basil Essential Oil

- In your diffuser, add 3 parts basil oil to 1 part peppermint oil. The aroma will instantly uplift your mood and revitalize your energy.

Top 3 Essential Oils for Balancing Hormones

Thyme Essential Oil

Thyme oil boosts the production of progesterone in the body. So how does this help? Well, low progesterone levels in the body have been linked to infertility, depression and PCOS (polycystic ovarian syndrome). There is a well-documented study about this in the *'Proceedings of the Society of Experimental Biology and Medicine'*. Because it is a natural hormone balancer, it is preferred by many people over synthetic hormone replacement therapies.

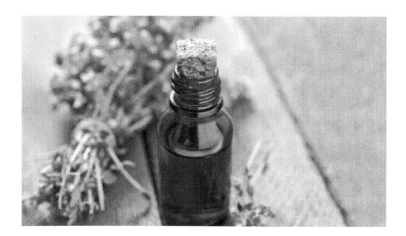

Clary Sage Essential Oil

Clary sage essential oil is another type of oil with significant benefits to the body in terms of hormone balance. It reduces cortisol levels in the body thereby alleviating stress. It also improves thyroid hormone levels and balances out estrogen production in the body. The dangers hormonal imbalance poses to the body are endless, and with clary sage essential oil, you can avoid conditions like PCOS, cancers, chronic stress and infertility.

How to Use Clary Sage and Thyme Essential Oils

- Add 20 to 30 drops of clary sage oil to 20 to 30 drops of thyme essential oil and blend it with an ounce of primrose oil. Store this blend in a dark glass container from which you will be rubbing about 5 drops around your neck twice every week.

Sandalwood Essential Oil

Sandalwood balances out testosterone levels in both men and women. It has also been found to be a natural aphrodisiac. You can improve your libido and balance out your T-hormones with this oil.

How to Use Sandalwood Essential Oil

- Mix some coconut oil with sandalwood oil and rub it on different parts of the body. This will allow them to be absorbed into the body through the skin.

Top 3 Essential Oils for Gut Health and Digestion

Oregano Essential Oil

Oregano oil contains potent antibacterial, anti-fungal and anti-parasitic healing compounds making it one of the most powerful essential oils for digestion. It has been found to kill off pathogenic gut bacteria that live in the digestive system. Its active compound is called carvacrol which kills yeast and other harmful bacteria. Because it is so strong, it is only recommended for use when in distress to get regular digestion back on track.

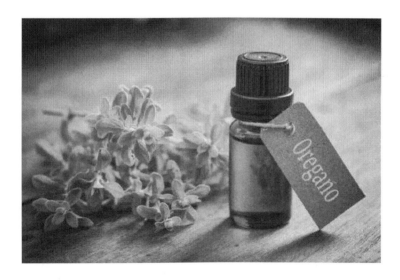

How to Use Oregano Oil

- For digestive issues or viral infections, dilute a drop of this oil in 500 ml of water and drink it (make sure to check with your doctor before doing this).

Peppermint Essential Oil

This is a fragrant, stimulating and refreshing type of oil that is widely used for digestive issues. It also eases common nausea, indigestion, and gas while stimulating your digestive process.

How to Use Peppermint Essential Oil

- Add a drop or two in a vegetarian gel capsule and take daily or as needed.
- You can also blend it with your pre-workout drink for an energizing start or wind down after your workout with your favorite shake.

The root of ginger has been used for centuries, and continues to be used, in kitchens all over the world for its ability to reduce symptoms of common stomach upset including nausea, bloating and gas. The oil extracted from it is used to stimulate digestion and sooth the gut.

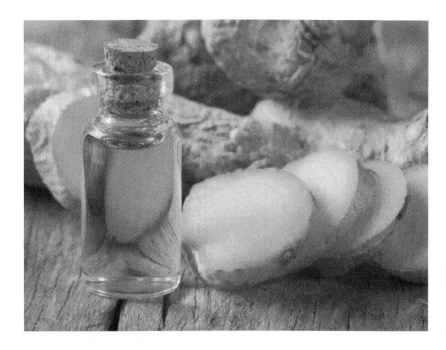

How to Use Ginger Essential Oil

- Inhale some directly out of the bottle or put some in your diffuser. The vapors carry active chemical molecules into your body through the nose. These chemicals stimulate your nasal cavity sending signals directly to your central nervous system – the system by which digestion is governed.

Top 3 Essential Oils for Headaches, Injury and Pain Management

Chamomile Essential Oil

Chamomile's analgesic properties are very useful when treating headaches and neuralgia, along with muscle and joint pains. It can also be used to relieve abdominal pain brought by bloating. While German Chamomile is preferred when handling inflammatory conditions, Roman Chamomile is ideal in soothing abdominal discomfort.

How to Use Chamomile Essential Oil

- Use chamomile oil with a diffuser or apply topically to the affected area after diluting with some carrier oil.

Eucalyptus Essential Oil

Eucalyptus oil is a powerful decongestant with anti-inflammatory properties that contribute to pain relief from sinus congestion and muscle injuries. It is quite strong; therefore, it should be diluted with some carrier oil when applying on the skin. You can use it raw when used to treat insect stings and bites.

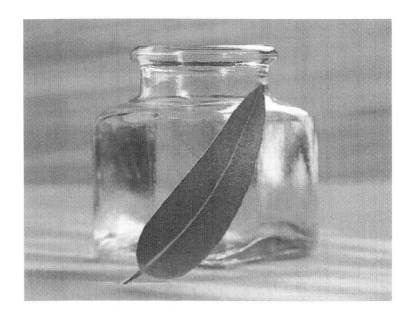

How to Use Eucalyptus Essential Oil

- Blend the oil with other Essential Oils such as Lavender to enhance its effects.
- Use in your bath water by dropping a few drops of the oil in it.
- You can also use as a lotion and rub it lightly on affected areas.

Peppermint Essential Oil

The highly refreshing smell of the oil comes from the active ingredient menthol – a major component of the oil. It has been used to relieve stomachaches, indigestion and nausea. When used topically, it relaxes muscles in the lower back, reduces tension headaches and pain due to fibromyalgia.

How to Use Peppermint Essential Oil

- Mix a few drops of this oil with a teaspoonful of some carrier oil. Apply the blend topically to the affected area, or the temples in case of a headache. Make sure the oil doesn't come in contact with your eyes.

Top 3 Essential Oils for Cleaning Your Home

Tea Tree Essential Oil

Tea tree oil is quite strong in killing germs, viruses and bacteria, and that is why it is a common ingredient in hand wipes and hand soaps. It can also be used as a bug repellant and an air freshener that gets rid of musty smells around your house. Not many essential oils have their antifungal and antiseptic properties off the charts quite like tea tree essential oil and for these reasons, it makes the list of the best oils for home cleaning.

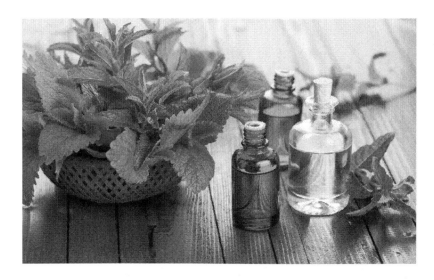

- Add a couple of teaspoons of this oil to two cups of water in a clean spray bottle to make a cleaner for moldy and dusty areas.
- Make a solution of water and mild soap and add a few drops of tea tree essential oil to it. Use the mixture to mop your floor.

Lemon Essential Oil

This oil is popular and preferred for its light and clean scent. Naturally antibacterial and antiviral, lemon is commonly used to degrease stubborn stains as well as make the air fresher for longer.

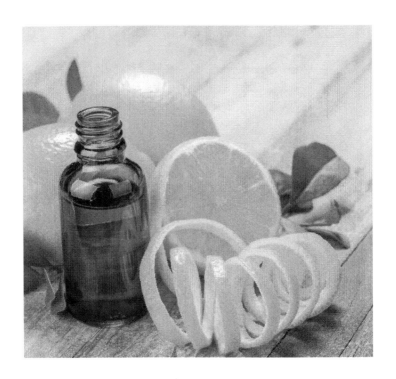

How to Use Lemon Essential Oil

- Lemon oil can be used in a myriad of different ways. You can combine it with olive oil to make for a natural wood or leather polish. You can mix it with other essential oils, such as lavender oil and tea tree oil, along with some alcohol, to make for a powerful house cleaning liquid.

- Add a few drops of this oil to your laundry detergent to brighten your white clothes and give them a fresh scent.

Wild Orange Essential Oil

Wild orange oil has many of the properties that lemon oil has with one of the few differences being that it has more of a 'happy' scent. It is a powerful grease remover, germ killer and air freshener. Just like lemon oil, wild orange oil also has a ton of uses and can be used both in combination with other oils or just by itself.

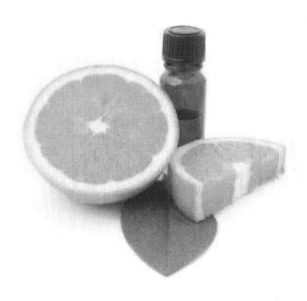

How to Use Wild Orange Oil

- Use a couple of drops to lift grease or glue from surfaces.
- Combine about a dozen drops with 1/4 cup castile soap and water to wipe down stovetops and counters.

Chapter 6: Fun with Oils

How to Use Essential Oils

Air Freshener Spray

It is hard to keep up with the number of home fragrance products available today. From scented sprays and oil diffusers to incense and plug-in room deodorizes, the industry has it all. The problem is that a lot of these products are filled with chemicals and toxins that are harmful to our bodies. A few drops of some highly concentrated essential oil can provide your home with the much needed sweet and fresh fragrance. For a homemade air freshener spray, all you need are: a clean empty spray bottle, some water, your favorite essential oil and a bit of undiluted alcohol such as vodka. The most commonly used essential oils in air fresheners sprays include: lavender, lemon, lime, rosemary, clary sage, clove and orange oils.

Bath Salts

You have probably heard of the soothing effects of a lavender essential oil bath or a peppermint essential oil bath. These baths offer a wonderful destressing, pain relieving, skin softening and relaxing feeling after a long hard day. These baths can also be used to treat bacterial infections. Oil and water do not mix; therefore, just adding some essential oil to your bath won't help much. In fact, if anything, it may irritate or burn your skin. You can mix it with a carrier oil first to negate the chances of irritation, but may still not mix properly with water. What people usually do is mix essential oil with some bath salts first so that it is able to fully disperse and infuse in the bath.

Add about 10 to 20 drops of oil, such as lavender or rosemary, to your favorite bath salts before infusing them in a water bath. The most common bath salts used with oils include: dead sea salt, Epsom salt and sea salt.

Candles

The idea behind burning scented candles is usually to eliminate foul odors in the room, create a more festive and welcoming atmosphere or for aromatherapy purposes such as uplifting the spirit and calming your mind. Making your own candles is as inexpensive as it is easy. These scented candles can also make for a good gift to your loved ones. Depending on the purpose you want to achieve, choose an essential oil that fits you. You can refer to the previous chapter in the uses of various oils.

Typically, the recommended ratio is an ounce of oil to a pound of wax but you can tweak it and see what works for you. It should be noted that since candles involve the oils coming into contact with direct heat, there is a possibility that you may get very little scent because the heat destroys the oils. Candles are not the most effective way to disperse wonderful fragrances around the house, but you can always try and see how it comes out.

Gel Sprays

Essential oils can provide a natural and cost-effective way to care for your dreadlocks. The most common blends being used today for gel sprays feature essential oils such as: tea tree oil, lavender oil, rosemary oil and peppermint oil mixed with a base such as Aloe Vera gel. Organic Aloe Vera is far better than its synthetic counterpart and it can be used to treat or relieve the following conditions.

- Burns
- Fungus
- Scalp itchiness
- Eczema
- As a hand sanitizer

Besides Aloe Vera, other bases used for making a DIY gel spray include: rich creams, lotions and heavy butters.

Humidifier

Diffusing essential oils in your house creates a pleasant scent, uplifts or calms your mood, cleanses the air, heals physical infirmities and balances emotions. Most diffusers use cold air to break down the particles of the essential oil which means the integrity of the oil is maintained. Humidifiers, on the other hand, use warm air which can damage the oil's particles thereby compromising its therapeutic properties. Also, because humidifiers run constantly, your body is not given the time to absorb the dispersed oil. Some essential oils such as citrus-based oils have been found to break down plastics, which can damage your humidifier in the long run. For these reasons it is not always advisable to use humidifiers to disperse essential oil.

Aromatherapy massage provides a remarkable synergy that not only relieves stress and tension, but also boosts the general well-being of someone. Custom massage oils are commonly made by combining essential oils and carrier oils. There are a million recipes available for aromatherapy massage oils. If scent is huge deal breaker for you, make a point of sampling scents of different essential oils and carrier oils first so that you can get a sense of what the finished product will smell like. When mixing oils, do it one step at a time and sample the resulting scent. Keep track of the quantities or ratios used so that you can replicate it in the future. The most popular carrier oils used for aromatherapy massage oils are: sweet almond oil, cold-pressed coconut oil, grapeseed oil, jojoba oil and olive oil.

Easy DIY Diffuser Blends You Can Make Yourself

Diffusing one type of oil is good enough but what's better? Diffusing a blend of different types of oils! The following are some popular blends you can put in your diffuser:

Rejuvenating Freshness

Step into summertime freshness with a scent that hits all your limbic system senses. This blend will fill your heart with peace and love. Combine 2 drops of spearmint oil, 2 drops of grapefruit oil, and 2 drops of lemon oil and 3 drops of lavender oil in your diffuser.

Dissolve the Stench

In a household setting, stench can come from filthy sports uniform, pet odors or even the trash can. A blend of 2 drops of lemon oil, 1 drop of tea tree oil, 1 drop of lime oil and 1 drop of cilantro oil can do wonders for your home.

Is It Allergy Season Again? No Problem

Seasonal allergies can make life really miserable – whether they come in the summer or winter. With a proper blend of essential oils, the effects of your allergies will be alleviated or kept at bay. Mix 3 drops of lemon oil and 3 drops of lavender oil with 3 drops of peppermint oil in your diffuser and begin to enjoy the allergy-relieving effects of this blend.

Eliminate the Bugs

Bugs like roaches, mosquitoes, ants and houseflies can really be a nuisance around the house. Bugs typically like to hide in places like: dark spots, corners, cracks in the wall, trash cans and under the sink. An ideal diffuser blend for this is made by combining 1 drop of lemongrass oil, 1 drop of basil oil, 1 drop of thyme oil and 1 drop of eucalyptus oil.

Goodnight Princess

After a long hard day, what you are often looking forward to is a good night's rest. Essential oils can do wonders for you in your journey into slumber land. Make a blend for your diffuser by mixing 2 drops of lavender oil, 2 drops of marjoram oil and 2 drops of chamomile for pleasant night.

Chapter 7: Frequently Asked Questions

How can I use essential oils on children?

Treat essential oils like medication by keeping them out of reach of children. Some like wintergreen can be very toxic in large doses while others like melaleuca are toxic even in small doses when taken internally. When using on kids, make sure you dilute them in carrier oils or in a bath as described in the packaging. If you have to apply them topically, do it to the bottom of their feet.

Which essential oils are safe to use when pregnant?

Pregnancies are very sensitive – especially during the first trimester because your baby develops rapidly at this stage. When pregnant, always dilute your oils before using them rather than applying them directly onto your skin. Where possible, use aromatherapy instead of ingesting or topical application. Essential oils to avoid when pregnant are: Basil, Cassia, Cinnamon, Clary Sage, Lemongrass, Rosemary, Thyme, Vetiver, Wintergreen and White Fir Oils.

Is it okay to use essential oils when breastfeeding?

Some essential oils, like peppermint oil, can decrease milk supply; therefore you should minimize their usage. The packaging found in the oils will usually contain guidelines on how and when to use essential oils when breastfeeding. Generally speaking, the following oils are considered safe to use when breastfeeding (but always check with your doctor first): Ylang Ylang, Wild Orange, Sandalwood, Roman Chamomile, Patchouli, Melaleuca, Lemon, Lavender, Geranium, Grapefruit, Clary Sage and Bergamot Oils.

How much should I use?

Most essential oils are very strong; so, as a general practice, always use a little since it will go a long way. Start with just one drop and work up from there, unless you have a recipe or suggested protocol that recommends doing otherwise.

Can I use more than one blend at a time?

Yes you can. Have fun and layer the blends freely to customize the combination of your individual needs. One blend can produce different results to different people. However, some blends don't make sense in combination; for example an Invigorate blend and a sleep blend.

If I'm allergic to the plant, can I still use its essential oil?

Yes, probably. Plant allergies are to the protein of the plant: the leaf, the seed, the pollen, etc. None of that is present in the essential oil. Do your own research (and consult your doctor) and do what you feel comfortable with. You can always try the oil in an inconspicuous location to see how you respond. If you do get a rash from using oil from a plant that you are allergic to, it doesn't necessarily mean that you are allergic to the oil. It could be because you applied too much or the dilution was not enough.

Is it safe to drink essential oils internally?

Yes and no. Something that is safe for one person may not be safe for another due to things like allergies, sensitivities, or contraindicated health issues. Before deciding to take any essential oil internally, check its quality, purity, and testing. Now, if you are still confused about all this, it is best to consult with your doctor before deciding to ingest any type of essential oil.

How should I store my essential oils and blends?

Keep your oils away from direct heat and light. Store them in a dark glass bottle and in a cool and dry area. When correctly stored, your oils can stay in good condition for up to 2 years. Ideally, the best place to store your aromatherapy oils is in a dry, dark room with a temperature slightly below 68 F. Also, only buy what you are going to be using. There's no need to buy more than enough.

What precautions should I take when using essential oils?

Essential oils have multiple uses and so precautions tend to vary depending on their usage. Also, most of these precautions are described in the packaging but I'll just go ahead and summarize some of them.

- ✓ Use high quality pure oils.
- ✓ When in doubt, dilute with some carrier oil.
- ✓ It is advisable to carry out a skin test before topical application of any oil.
- ✓ Keep them out of reach of your eyes.
- ✓ In case of skin irritation, stop using the oil. If you're using it concentrated, try diluting it before using it again.

How do I tell the right blend for me?

Blend is all about what you need and what you like. If blends seem similar, try them both to see which one fits you best. Choose blends based on what they can do for you.

Bonus

Essential Oil Salad Recipes

French Cucumber Salad infused with Marjoram Essential Oil

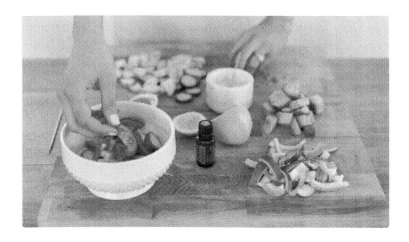

Ingredients

- 2 toothpicks of Marjoram essential oil
- 2 tomatoes, diced
- 2 whole avocados, diced
- 2 tablespoons of olive oil
- Salt to taste
- ¾ red onion, sliced
- 1 whole cucumber, diced
- 2 tablespoons of freshly squeezed lemon juice

Method

1. In a large bowl, mix together the avocado, tomatoes, red onions and cucumber.
2. Pour olive oil into the mixture along with Marjoram essential oil
3. Add some lemon juice and salt to taste.
4. Lightly mix the ingredients once more and serve immediately.

Lemon Essential Oil Vinaigrette Salad Dressing

Ingredients

- 3 drops of Lemon Essential Oil
- Salt to taste
- 1 teaspoon of ground mustard
- 3 tablespoons of apple cider vinegar
- 2 teaspoons of pure honey
- 2 tablespoons of grated onion
- 5 tablespoons of extra virgin olive oil

Method

1. In a small bowl, combine all the ingredients together and whisk until they are well combined.
2. Pour this dressing over a variety of your favorite salads. It works well with chicken salad, tuna salad and fruit salads.

Kale Caesar Salad with Wild Orange Essential Oil Dressing

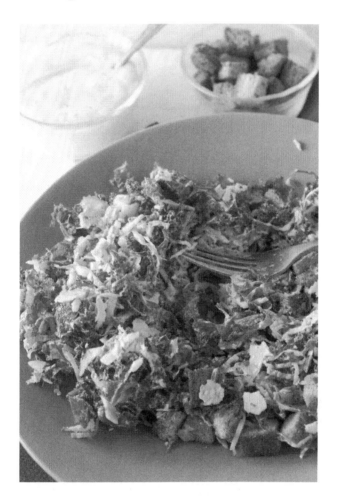

Ingredients

- A large bunch of curly kale

- A cup of sunflower seeds some of which will be used for garnish
- Sea salt to taste
- A slice of crusty bread
- 2 cloves of garlic
- 2 to 3 drops of Wild Orange Essential Oil
- ¾ cup of raw almonds, activated
- ½ teaspoon of smoked paprika
- ¼ teaspoon of chili powder
- 1¼ cups of distilled water
- 1½ teaspoons of rice malt syrup
- Parmesan cheese sprinkle

Method

1. Rinse the kale leaves and pat dry with a paper towel before cutting it up into bite size pieces and place them in a bowl.
2. Combine all the other ingredients in a blender and blend until they are nice, smooth and creamy.
3. Pour half the mixture over the kale in the bowl and mix until all of it is coated.

4. Add the remaining mixture and work it well into the kale and let it rest for 10 minutes to tenderize the leaves.

5. Plate the greens and garnish with some sunflower seeds to your satisfaction

Conclusion

You now understand that essential oils are a must have in your home. You can use them for hygiene purposes, general well-being or for mental and spiritual health. Thanks to the information provided in this book, you can start making your own custom blends and still find ways to introduce these oils to your daily diet. You have all the right tools and information to find a trustworthy and reliable essential oils dealer and are able to use these oils responsibly to benefit both yourself and your loved ones. Enjoy!

Manufactured by Amazon.ca
Bolton, ON

32754427R00074